Table of Contents

An In-Depth Exploration of Steroids for Treating Back Pain

1. Introduction to Back Pain and Steroids

1.1. Overview of Back Pain

1.2. Types of Steroids Used

2. Mechanism of Action

2.1. Anti-Inflammatory Properties

2.2. Pain-Relief Mechanisms

3. Efficacy and Effectiveness

3.1. Clinical Studies and Evidence

4. Administration Methods

4.1. Oral Steroids

4.2. Epidural Steroid Injections

5. Potential Side Effects

5.1. Short-Term Side Effects

5.2. Long-Term Side Effects

6. Patient Considerations and Counseling

6.1. Patient Selection Criteria

6.2. Precautions and Monitoring

7. Comparative Analysis with Other Treatments

7.1. Physical Therapy

7.2. Surgical Interventions

8. Future Research and Developments

8.1. Emerging Trends in Steroid Use

An In-Depth Exploration of Steroids for Treating Back Pain

1. Introduction to Back Pain and Steroids

The Global Burden of Disease Study 2019 reported that the population prevalence of low back pain was 5779 per 100,000 individuals. This condition has been shown to have wide-ranging social and psychological impacts, including high levels of morbidity, the loss of workdays as a result of pain-related disability, and can also have a number of economic consequences. Furthermore, the condition eludes accurate identification, with the cause of the majority of lower back pain cases not specifically identifiable☐ hence the treatment options for these cases are even more complex. Steroids, or corticosteroids, are commonly used in medicine to combat inflammation or act as an adjuvant therapy, with options for oral, rectal, topical, locally injected, or intravenously administered steroids. When used to manage low back pain, steroids are most often used where a clear inflammation focus (e.g., lumbar radicular herniation) is evidenced by findings.

This essay will take a comprehensive approach to examining the use of steroids in treating back pain. This is an appropriate topic, given that back pain is a common and highly debilitating health condition affecting a wide swathe of the general population. It has been highlighted by a number of clinical studies as a favorable means of treating inflammation which may underpin some of the causes of this condition. However, concerns have been expressed about the development of side effects associated with their administration, and wider questions have been raised regarding their effectiveness.

Introduction

1.1. Overview of Back Pain

Assuming blood tests, magnetic resonance imaging, and x-rays continue to be unproductive, clinical guidelines for well-established spinal injections show that proper long-term pain relief was acquired with gabapentinoids and graded exercise. Despite the fact that there is no agreement on how back pain could be treated, certain guidance has said that for individuals experiencing acute and continual lower back pain, first-line therapy entails analgesics and non-steroidal anti-inflammatory drugs. Opioids are an alternative in pain relief, although they have been associated with potential complications and addictive behavior. A handful of co-interventions are an alternative to the immediate termination of opioid therapy. One of the biologic interventions proposed is the injection of corticosteroids and anesthetic, which can potentially be performed at the trigger points, facet joints, sacroiliac joints, epidural space, as well as intradiscal, and as undirected nerve blocks.

An important part of our country's healthcare work is treating back pain. Back pain is often viewed as a symptom of some sort of underlying damage. It is estimated that about 84% of North Americans will suffer from severe back pain during their lives. Back pain can occur from numerous sources, such as conditions, mechanical or degenerative lesions, infection, and malignant disease. It can also be divided into acute, subacute, or chronic kind based upon the degree of pain and the length of recurrence.

1.2. Types of Steroids Used

Corticosteroids are hormone-like compounds produced by the adrenal glands (small glands located above the kidneys) as part of the body's natural stress and inflammatory responses. Because they are so effective for rapidly relieving pain or dramatically reducing local inflammation, corticosteroids are often used medically both to modulate the body's immune system (e.g. in autoimmune conditions like rheumatoid arthritis or Crohn's Disease) and to shrink swollen tissue (e.g. in the brain after a traumatic injury). Clinicians choose between corticosteroids for injection based primarily on their anti-inflammatory versus mineralocorticoid effects (side effects they may produce). Anabolic steroids, by contrast, are compounds designed to mimic certain hormone effects produced by the male gonads and adrenal glands. They are not synthetic versions of corticosteroids, and they are not used medically in anesthesiology and pain management, which is the primary focus of this review.

In the treatment of low back pain, several different types of steroids are used. Generally, steroids used in the treatment of back pain are classified as either corticosteroids or anabolic steroids. Specific examples of corticosteroids commonly injected for back pain include triamcinolone, betamethasone, dexamethasone, hydrocortisone, and methylprednisolone. Anabolic steroid mixtures are not typically used in the treatment of back pain.

2. Mechanism of Action

Most discs can cause this kind of pain effectively the bottom one-third to almost one-third of the body. Part of a spinal nerve is rooted by a mixture of sciatic and plexus nerves. Similar spinal nerve injection, unless prior steps are taken to achieve the actual root site (for example, injection results surrounding the nerve structures), laminar approach is performed, precisely introducing the tip of the needle with the aid of X-ray imaging into the key portion and mid-portion of the posterior spine disc. An intradiscal steroid injection can help decrease inflammation, which is often considered a large component of most back pain. Nerves can become compressed, leading patients to feel muscle tightness and discomfort. Inflammation is caused by chemicals secreted by injured tissue in response to the damage that results in nerve irritation, swelling, and the creation of scar tissue. Steroid medication can help to relieve inflammation, in addition to providing general pain relief.

An intradiscal steroid injection utilizes a corticosteroid medication combined with a local anesthetic. The injection is introduced into the middle of the spinal disc, which appears to be the origin of most of the sources of back pain. Although the prevalence of this type of injection can vary widely by area, up to 8% of all epidural steroid injections are thought to be intradiscal. Commonly, epidural nerve block steroids are used to offer pain relief and lower inflammation in some manner. Pain relief is obtained because they have steroid properties, which reduce inflammation as mentioned above, and local anesthetic characteristics, which block nerve impulses.

2.1. Anti-Inflammatory Properties

Steroids have established an outstanding status regarding their remarkable ability to modulate inflammatory response. In other words, steroids taken can decrease the patient's inflammation and pain. The level of the condition's entry influences its mod employees and the signs of swelling. However, it is considered healthy to have a modulated, symptomatic amount and inadequate for living in everyday life. This includes the Cephalic Zone, of which it is partly viral and partly-mediated subject.

Steroids, in their many forms, are naturally produced in the body in order to kill inflammation. For severe back pain, they can be greatly beneficial because dosage is given to constrain back pain, i.e., a symptomatic inflammation component. The inflammation's initial cause depends on whether or not steroids treat it. Cortisol is a part of our central nervous system's natural steroids.

For people suffering from severe back pain, they often turn to steroids. This article aims to flesh out the idea of steroids as pain management. It is thus dedicated to exploring the different facets of steroids and how they help battle neurological back pain. As such, a detailed overview of what steroids are is first provided. This is then followed by a discussion of the relevance of steroids due to their anti-inflammatory properties. The mechanism for such anti-inflammatory response is also unraveled. Finally, the principle of mitigation is then expanded upon.

2.2. Pain-Relief Mechanisms

Several researchers report that the analgesic effect of corticosteroids is related to a more rapid decrease in inflammation, as evidenced by a faster regression of edema and noticeable relief of pain. The mechanism by which corticosteroids reduce edema is not clear, although several actions have been proposed: corticosteroids may decrease the amount of fluid and synovial exudate in soft tissue by inhibiting the deposition of neutrophils and fibrin; or they may reduce intracapsular inflammation and edema and decompress fine terminal nerve branches within periarticular connective tissues. De Schoot et al. (1994) attribute the short-term beneficial analgesic effect of corticosteroids to multiple effects on several levels of the nociceptive system and state that it seems to be mediated as much centrally as peripherally. Steroidal anti-inflammatory agents in the epidural space can result in pain relief with both a rapid and delayed onset, according to studies. More recent reports suggest that steroids also have an effect on the dorsal horn of neurons in the spinal cord, mostly at the level of A-beta fibers. Steroids have an anti-inflammatory effect at the injured part of the spine. Even a single steroid injection has a positive long-term effect by impairing intra-articular tissue metabolism and preventing inflammation. Opioid release, efficiency of local anesthetic action, inhibition of phospholipase A2, and a metabolic cascade all could contribute to this beneficial effect. In traditional medicine, oral steroids are often given on a dosing schedule known as a tapered dose pack, beginning with a high dosage and decreasing by a certain percentage with each previous dosage. For this treatment of back pain, no specific program has been determined. The dosage of steroid varies depending on the doctor's preference, but it is a reasonable close ratio. Furthermore, some other dosing options are recommended, including moderate, high, and very high injectables as well as treatments in which the injectable is delivered through two levels. Moreover, there is a wide range of dosage options for steroid injections. It is important to note that current studies do not fully support the use of large dosing. Furthermore, including dosing charts with both weight- and concentration-based efficacy from major steroid vendors in eosinophilic esophagitis is dishonest and controversial. At this time, many physicians recommend using the highest dose that still has a defined safety maximum (e.g., 12ml). It is worth noting that a higher steroid dose does not always yield better results.

Steroids reduce swelling and edema throughout the body, including inflamed disc material, which reduces the pressure inside the disk or on the adjacent nerve. This action will decrease nerve root "cross talk," as well. Use of steroids in the epidural space can result in systemic delivery and provide whole body relief. There are steroid receptors in several locations in the body, including the central and peripheral nervous system. The receptors, when activated or blocked by a steroid, promote a cascade of cellular events, which can ultimately influence many metabolic pathways. Steroids can block inflammation and the acute immune response. They can open the bronchial airways in the lungs. They can alter the metabolism of carbohydrates, protein, and fat. They can stabilize lysosomal membranes and prevent further release of cell wall-destroying enzymes. In addition, the basal vasoconstrictive tone (constriction of blood vessels) that is increased by excess levels of lactic acid is reduced. Steroids also block the release of many pain-producing substances from damaged or inflamed tissues.

3. Efficacy and Effectiveness

Clinical studies show that corticosteroids are an effective and safe treatment for low back pain, radiculopathy (which defines spinal nerve roots), and sciatica. There is evidence suggesting that local corticosteroid injections can reduce pain in some patients with persistent local pressure symptoms and reduction of active treatment. Although drugs have a potent analgesic effect, even in the presence of enhanced inflammation, wearing off the drug after corticosteroid injection in traumatic plantar fasciitis and low-dose application of chronic muscle relaxation - both in patients with dorsal lumbar spinal stenosis - are not only common, but also principal. The evidence supporting the effectiveness of long-term oral systemic corticosteroids as a treatment option is modest.

It is suggested that trials put greater emphasis on effectiveness of the intervention rather than just being concerned with efficacy, and it is recommended to introduce the new term "efficacyplus". Offering a drug as a proven solution to pain should be based on solid evidence, as increasing the number of reporting unethical cases is possibly due to rising insurance costs caused by the use of the term "efficacy" in marketing strategies.

3.1. Clinical Studies and Evidence

More recently, Armon et al. conducted a network meta-analysis on epidural steroid injections compared to other treatments for sciatica. They found 38 studies in the clinical literature with 11 different comparisons, many of which had limited data upon which to draw conclusions. They found that evidence for interlaminar injections of steroids showed "a medium-significant advantage...[at] 3 and 6 weeks follow-up." There are two things to bear in mind when reading this evidence. First and foremost, "low back pain" is a term that encompasses a myriad of different types and etiologies. Exceptional rigor is therefore required when designing, conducting, and interpreting a clinical trial on low back pain. Does a steroid shot help a patient who just recently injured his or her back while lifting weights? Does it help someone with back pain due to ankylosing spondylitis? There is no reason to think that a steroid shot would be useful in both scenarios.

So what does the data in the clinical literature show? Koes et al. conducted a systematic review and meta-analysis of randomized control trials evaluating the efficacy of epidural corticosteroid injections. They found 25 trials that met their inclusion criteria. They concluded that "previous results of one positive high quality trial and seven positive low quality trials could be explained by publication bias. Insufficient or no evidence was found for long-term pain relief and for improvement in back-specific functional status in patients with low back pain."

4. Administration Methods

4.2. Epidural steroid injections (ESI) for back pain Back pain can be treated with a variety of treatment options, including spine, back, or neck pain, and interventional pain management treatment. This procedure involves incorporating a safe epidural injection into the epidural space in the vertebral column that encompasses the cerebrospinal fluid, nerves, blood vessels, meninges, and fat. The course of intervention must ensure strict aseptic precautions are being observed. After delivery, the steroids begin to operate by decreasing inflammation and reducing pain, and some people may experience a slowing or halting of the progress of the disease. The current guidelines for lumbar intervertebral disc herniation-associated pain from previous epidural steroid injection strongly suggest lumbar microdiscectomy for persistent radiculopathy. However, three recent studies suggest ESI without a subsequent surgical procedure is responsible for relief, particularly short-term benefit in pain and function, in patients suffering from acute radiculopathy.

4.1. Oral steroids for back pain Oral corticosteroids are more commonly used to relieve pain and inflammation in many health issues. They involve steroids such as glucocorticoids that are designed to work like cortisol, but administered orally. Medicines featuring glucocorticoids include Prednisolone and Prednisone. Dexamethasone is another steroid medication prescribed to reduce severe inflammation due to many conditions, including hormone disorders and certain forms of arthritis. Prednisone is often used to ease inflammation and pain caused by different forms of arthritis and other conditions. There is also a delayed-release prednisone medication that aims to reduce pain and swelling. Oral steroids have two modalities of use in back pain sufferers. Short-term pain relief is for patients who require rapid improvement of symptoms, and long-term for patients who require slow symptom control, especially those used in patients awaiting elective decompression surgery. This drug is also administered for conditions such as meningitis, allergies, multiple sclerosis, and asthma.

4.1. Oral Steroids

The dosing can be adjusted for individual circumstances and the patient's weight. However, if someone is significantly overweight, the steroid may not be as effective, as one ophthalmological paper suggests. The reasoning behind corticosteroids typically only working if the person weighs 120 kg (265 lbs) or less is not addressed. Often, though, oral steroids are taken considering the side effect profile and the duration of therapy as being much less significant than with an epidural space, intramuscular, or intravenous steroids. Some physician offices will give an injection of one's choice, immediately following an appointment for care, to reinforce the effects of IM corticosteroids.

Administering oral steroids is the easiest and most common way of using corticosteroids. Most commonly, a healthcare provider will prescribe a "MethylPrednisolone Dose Pack" if a patient has typically been responsive to using them for treating various types of pain. We use low-dose Medrol Dosepacks in the clinic. The dosing typically includes 6 doses on the first day, 5 on the next, 4 doses on the third day, and so forth, to give a short initial burst that typically reduces or halts inflammation quickly. The script (i.e., prescription) is typically provided for a 6- or 12-day burst. It is common in musculoskeletal medicine to use a six-day "Dose Pack," but we prefer the 12-day pack if the patient can tolerate the medication. The oral steroids are then tapered toward the end of their use. If the patient discontinues the medicine before they have been on it for a minimum of 12 days, it is unlikely that they received a significant anti-inflammatory or tissue repairing value from it.

4. Steroids for treating back pain 4.1. Oral steroids

4.2. Epidural Steroid Injections

Key clinical considerations include the use of particulate (versus non-particulate) steroids and which steroids to choose. When a particulate steroid is used, position the bevel of the needle towards the outside of the sac, as to keep the medication near the pathology that is causing the pain. Alternatively, a position toward the inside of the sac is used when one administers non-particulate steroids. As for which steroids to choose, certain practitioners prefer dexamethasone over other drugs, thought to be due to its longer duration of action. Finally, inter-laminar epidural injections tend to provide pain relief to broader-based pathology but also have higher rates of dural puncture as a potential complication.

As mentioned before, steroids have proven to be a useful treatment for various back-related conditions, including disc herniations, degenerative disc disease, discogenic pain, spinal stenosis, and spondylolisthesis. While the previous instances of steroid administration have investigated oral Medrol dose packs and intramuscular depot preparations, there is enhanced efficacy in injecting steroids directly into the epidural space. This method targets the site of inflammation and, theoretically, should produce faster results with lower side effects. Alternative approaches can be taken with the epidural injection, including inter-laminar, transforaminal (caudal or inter-laminar), and transfacet approaches. Data suggest a longer pain-free interval with the transforaminal technique, the most commonly used method for many physiatrists, while the inter-laminar technique is the most commonly used in the remainder of the world.

5. Potential Side Effects

Long-term adverse events: Regular corticosteroids can have negative effects on many body systems. Steroid injections can cause pseudoseptic arthritis or a steroid flare following an injection, with pain and redness at the injection site. Overall, up to 3% of all patients may experience a long-term adverse outcome. Fully 2 people out of 50 undergoing spinal injection therapy are likely to have side effects that prove to be severe, primarily owing to the rarity of events with low background frequencies in this cross-sectional investigation.

Short-term adverse events: Anabolic or performance-enhancing steroids are manufactured substances that resemble the body's natural hormones. A treatment applying small amounts of corticosteroids into the epidural space (the area around the spinal cord) provides benefits for specific spinal conditions, such as sciatica, spinal stenosis, and herniated disc. Most likely, patients receive epidural steroids to suppress cytokines and chemokines in the epidural space, and researchers' hypothesis that these inflammatory mediators may be linked to herniated disc-induced sciatica. Steroid medications cause immediate effects on the central nervous system, which can lead to elevated blood pressure, rapid heart rate, nervousness, sleep disturbance, and loss of appetite.

General effects of steroids: The synthesis of this clinical practice guideline was prompted by the increasing frequency of a patient using anabolic or corticosteroids.

Both come from the common parent compound, cholesterol, and thus share profound effects on the human body, particularly at the cellular level. Over 150 anabolic steroids are currently registered for therapeutic use in the United States as medications to treat a variety of indications. Although anabolic and corticosteroids share a common biologic precursor, they are fundamentally different in regards to their effects and characteristics. Anabolic or performance-enhancing steroids are manmade substances related to male sex hormones. Men and women are more likely to experience short-term adverse events following steroid administration than prolonged ones, and the frequency of patients experiencing adverse events increases as follow-up extends from 4 months to 2 years. An exploratory subgroup analysis showed that the frequency of experiencing an adverse event related to steroid administration is higher for patients following lumbar steroid administration than it is for those receiving cervical injections.

5.1. Short-Term Side Effects

Side effects from using steroids are undesirable manifestations that arise from the action of steroids in therapy. These consequences may be of relevance to an athlete taking steroids, but would also be of concern when a clinician is considering giving steroids as a treatment option. In the clinical setting, side effects may occur and usually involve transient pain at the site of the injection. For example, a subcutaneous pad of fat (i.e., adipose) is found between the skin and the long bone of the thigh bone (or femur), which is called the greater trochanter. Nonetheless, a person who receives an injection of steroids directly to the greater trochanter could experience a mild-to-severe anamnesis, accompanied by tenderness. This could potentially lead to a diagnosis of having a disease called avascular necrosis, which of necessity would restrict physical activity, generally making daily life more challenging.

In Epidural steroid injections: A comprehensive review, authors provide a survey of the efficacy and safety of epidural steroid injections (ESIs) administered for treating low back and radicular leg pain. The primary review purpose, as described by the authors, was to deliberate the benefits and risks of using ESIs in the aforementioned clinical setting. Segmenting the analysis into ESIs for unilateral lumbar radiculopathy and bilateral pain (in separate sections), the authors first consider relevant patient outcomes (e.g., pain, disability), comparing patients worldwide who received an operative orchestration and

ESIs (treated) to patients across the globe who had only undergone the aforementioned operative procedure (untreated). At study conclusion, the authors found that among anti-edema benefits and the capability of ESIs to produce an intracanalological effect, complications clearly exist. In examining the reviewed studies, the authors assert that both treated and untreated patients achieved similar outcomes, suggesting that the wider application of ESIs would be imprudent because the need for proof of a treatment's worth is substantial. Once more, although ESIs can have proper short-term credentials, their identified complications must be considered.

5.2. Long-Term Side Effects

Some of the potential long-term side effects of the use of corticosteroid administration include immunosuppression, osteoporosis, avascular necrosis of bone, cataracts, insulin resistance, psychosis, diabetes, weight gain, and it can increase the need for surgical intervention in the back. Most of these disadvantages are associated with the repeated use of corticosteroids, suggesting that the more often a patient requires injections, the higher the risk of complications. By understanding these consequences, it becomes clear that the use of corticosteroids in the back should not be taken lightly and that its side effects and chronic potential should be more thoroughly examined to allow for more cautious treatment planning.

When treating patients who are suffering from lower back pain, particularly if the pain is not responding to other nonsurgical options, a common treatment for managing back pain has become the use of steroids. In some cases, this technique can help patients manage the pain. Furthermore, the injection of steroids helps to reduce the local inflammation of the spinal nerves, thus alleviating pain or discomfort. However, while the use of steroids appears, in the short term, particularly through clinical trials, to be beneficial, the evidence supporting its long-term impact is more limited. This criticism is supported by the outcome of the literature review, which pointed out that the effect of corticosteroids over time, particularly after repeated use, which can have serious consequences, deserves more comprehensive investigation.

6. Patient Considerations and Counseling

In the diabetic population, there has been some thought that an increased risk of retinal vein occlusions can result from peribulbar, intraorbital injections, as well as injections more remotely administered for other pain complaints in the head and neck. Risk management strategies of this nature have not been studied in the lumbar spine, but practitioners may want to be careful when considering the use of steroids to manage back pain in anyone with a substantially increased risk of retinal vein occlusion when additional procedures might also be indicated or should be considered. Steroids are often used to suppress the immune system. Consequently, an elevated risk of systemic infection from uncontrolled diabetes often necessitates that a patient schedule surgery to address potential sources of infection before receiving a steroid injection. A urinalysis may also be helpful in patients who are unable to sense urinary tract pain, as this could indicate a catheterized infection. Bacteremia, particularly from oral flora, is also a real risk. Although reports in the literature are limited, it is reasonable to assume that there could be a heightened risk for infection related to urinary incontinence if the sacral foramen are opened. Some experts argue that pertinent guidelines require the use of steroids to be discontinued in the three months prior to receiving a live attenuated vaccine. Electrification of the sacroiliac joint. This should be carefully discussed with the patient. Safety and efficacy data in patients who may have life-threatening allergic responses are sparse. A plan for rescue therapy should also be established if initial strategies fail. Steroid injections can have drug-drug interactions as well, so a thorough review of medications should be made. Close monitoring and intervention if an unwanted effect surfaces is also warranted. Beyond that, patients should be given pre-procedural counseling concerning back pain and the therapeutics that can be employed; factors including the potential for only short-lived pain relief should be clearly delineated. Outcomes in pain relief as reported in the literature and the need to modernize pain procedures with outcomes based on function and metrics other than pain scales alone should also be addressed.

Patient considerations and counseling are of paramount importance. In certain populations, epidural steroid injections are either not indicated or are considered high risk. In pregnant patients, the potential risks to the fetus can far outweigh the potential benefits. Steroids administered caudally in the lumbosacral region can quickly make their way into the systemic circulation and potentially cross the placenta. Some women will request this procedure for pain control. Counseling in advance by an obstetrician can help ensure treatment plans with which all parties are comfortable.

6.1. Patient Selection Criteria

The assessment of who has the potential to benefit from steroids is consecrated to be upon message for the consideration of cost-utility estimates/place in the care pathway for diabetes or low back pain pathway evaluation criteria. With a positive assessment, steroids can be cost-effective as a second-line intervention and clinically more effective in surgery compared with compounded pain-reducing medications (compounding use is considered experimental and used less across the UK, ranging from 4-18%) or to continue use. Those using steroids in surgery are clinically better and cost-effective. However, in negative scenarios, steroid therapy probably does not warrant the current ongoing use until evidence otherwise indicates how and when it should be used or that it does not provide added benefits. In patients that can potentially attain a benefit, two out of four do not use long-term opioids with true potential benefit as the short-term use under these criteria will avoid the use of long-term opioids.

Patient selection criteria: Prior to undertaking an effective treatment approach, clinicians deem it imperative to first elucidate the characteristics best suited for therapeutic steroids. A guideline compiled by the American Academy of Neurology enunciates a shared bond amongst all such patients by defining them as individuals with no overt malignancy, no infections, and no corresponding allergies to corticosteroids. As such, the parameters necessary for selecting the appropriate therapeutic steroids should be defined based on the root etiology of the low back pain.

However, prior to undertaking the administration of steroids, it is incumbent upon clinicians to first ensure patient relief via any one of the other non-invasive therapies. The assessment of these non-invasive therapies can be achieved by means of the Piercy rule - specifically, after a minimum of 1 to 4 weeks of the latest treatment, the co-occurrence of pain relief and improvement in functional abilities is scaled as the categorical fervency of the patient to undertake therapeutic steroids.

6.2. Precautions and Monitoring

Consult manufacturers' package inserts and SPCs (summaries of product characteristics) before performing any intervention. It is the responsibility of the clinician performing the procedure to be aware of the risks of the procedure, to communicate these to the patient, and to obtain valid, informed consent from the patient. Patients' cardiovascular status should be reviewed and optimized before considering steroid injection. Coagulation should be optimized in the presence of lady image findings (such as large disc herniation), which could represent a surgical emergency. Smaller image-defined lesions require a history of previous failure of conservative management with confirmed imaging findings correlating with the history. Intra-articular injection should be avoided in the presence of moderate or any sign of inflammation, sepsis, local malignancy, or deformity reducing the joint space. All the facts must be confirmed with imaging. Systemic sepsis is an absolute contraindication. HIAA axial spondyloarthritis must have both positive Japanese classification criteria and MRI positive findings.

• Use of aspiration by a small bore needle may be helpful in order to avoid unintentional intravascular injection of steroids. • Radiopaque steroid preparations may be helpful to demonstrate the spread despite non-intentional dural puncture. • Consider pre-7th day adrenal axis suppression testing in patients who are considered for repeat neuraxial steroid therapy. • The joint faculties of the Royal College of Anaesthetists (RCOA) and the Spinal Intervention Society support these statements. • A hyperglycemic management plan should be discussed if a patient receiving neuraxial steroid injections is found to have asymptomatic hyperglycemia. • There is insufficient evidence to support stopping anti-platelet agents to undertake epidural steroid injections (including transforaminal epidural steroid injections).

7. Comparative Analysis with Other Treatments

There are limited data comparing steroid injection to other non-pain-related therapies (e.g., physical therapy, surgery). There may be little or no difference in the effect of steroid injection on back pain, leg swelling, and disability compared to other treatments at early time points, such as physical therapy exercise, percutaneous discectomy (a discectomy carried out through the skin, not an incision), and block. Leg pain is likely more common or more extreme for patients who obtained a steroid injection than for those who received suction decompression. The effectiveness of skin discoloration coupled with advice and exercise compared to steroid injection, including skin color and advice, is also unknown for patients with back pain.

The use of steroids as an intervention to treat back pain is successful in relieving pain quickly. The long-term effects of this approach remain largely unclear, and additional research is required to increase the quality and generalizability of existing evidence. To control back pain through the use of steroids, numerous trials and studies have been conducted. Steroids have been injected, given with tablets, or applied as creams to provide pain relief. The use of such steroids has no high-level, long-term effects and is generally inconclusive. Therefore, further evidence is needed to ensure that the evidence produced is applicable to the general public and can be used to increase the confidence of healthcare practitioners. Whether a steroid should be used is also determined by a patient's symptom improvement, activity, or participation.

7.1. Physical Therapy

According to recent information, less than 5% of low back pain patients actually require surgery. Pandit et al cite in their US triage directory that less than 3% of patient initial evaluations predict a requirement for a specialist evaluation, whereas 80% of patients seen in primary care facilities have low back pain. Statistics suggest education has made a positive impact on implementation of guidelines toward addressing the recent opioid crisis. Most physicians currently will offer patients ibuprofen (NSAID), muscle relaxers, and OTC medications before prescribing opioids to apply to the recent CDC guidelines. There are currently three steroidal epidurals—Kenalog (a crystalline form of triamcinolone acetonide), Depo-Medrol (methylprednisolone acetate), and Celestone—a form of Betamethasone that cause water and sodium retention in the body, leading to an increase in high blood pressure.

Niazi et al. discussed alternate modalities toward managing patients with back pain. As part of an integrative approach to the patient, these options include soft tissue modality using Graston Technique and therapeutic exercises. It is the purpose of this discussion to explore the differences involved in medicating patients with steroids versus treating patients with therapeutic exercise using physical therapists.

7.2. Surgical Interventions

Not everyone is a good candidate for surgery or to receive steroid injections, and image-guided treatments such as these also increase the costs to society. Investigation would remain extremely multifaceted: 1. Extra time is involved. In the studies evaluated in this review, a multi-disciplinary panel discussed and proposed a consensus with surgical and interventional experts in attendance, following submission of cases with all non-invasive treatments exhausted. The panel deliberated and the final treatment was endorsed or otherwise. This review benefited greatly from the detailed methodological steps described within the included studies. However, there are some limitations of the current review.

Up until this point, this essay has looked almost exclusively at the use of steroids as a means to manage or treat symptoms of back pain. However, it is important to take surgical interventions as a point of comparison. Surgery has a unique advantage of providing an opportunity for the surgeon to aim directly at whatever they consider to be the cause of the pain, regardless of whether evidence exists to support a particular intervention philosophically. Both disc surgery and decompressions have been evaluated in our review for lumbar pain. Currently, there is one trial overview for radicular pain, but it has not been in a position to provide summary statistics. The difference between the two surgical interventions can be quite subtle and could be considered as two subgroups amongst those receiving 'surgical care'.

8. Future Research and Developments

The future research challenge is to clarify which subgroups have a positive response to steroid horrors. Pathways seek to determine the mechanism of Korean entrapment in small, randomized, blinded multi-arm trials. It seems strange that Chinese physicians are indeed science-oriented in this patient population, and those "classic" non-steroidal drugs are commonly used in the practice of other pain doctors. If rhIL-6 is the target, on the mitochondria vs. the cell membrane and the resulting neuroinflammation, future studies may have to examine local steroid vs. salsalate. Steroids that have been used for spinal injections need not be linked to politics. The next step is to study patients with back pain and leg pain separately from the US neuron-fascial syndrome. Bony/intraforaminal spinal lipoma, clinical factors as predictors of improvement, and four months of long-term functional testing and Extended Pain Reduction from Thoracic Spine Golf Transarticular Face $8 vs Interstitial No Change Glial Encasement Tumor Antagonist + prostaglandin 2 now with tranexamic acid.

In conclusion, a number of steroid trials now question the role of steroids, including thoracic transforaminal epidurals with contrast and particulates for discogenic pain. Although once thoracic discography was thought to have no benefit - financial, practical, or in terms of weak correlation with psychosocial form of care - a few recent articles, including reliable numbers of subjects, have moved in the direction of clinically relevant positive diagnostic studies of the thoracic spine. Although applying a highly sensitive reference standard due to the level of peripheral to central pain control, intradiscal injection of chromic copper in lumbosacral discography is still possibly an active research area. Yildiz unilaterally studied the technique in 20 patients with disc herniation who were not improved by physical therapy; 70% of patients improved by visual analog scale at 21 months of yolk. Research has shown that serial MRI follow-up and T2 mapping following MSC injection can discern MSC cell restoration from a fiberboard. Decreased fatty/collagen T2 macromolecules coincide with pain reduction after injection and lead to the hypothesis that T2 signal quantification could clarify the relationship between pain and grading on MRI.

8.1. Emerging Trends in Steroid Use

Nonsteroidal anti-inflammatory drugs (NSAIDs), a nonsteroidal anti-inflammatory drug (NSAID) which inhibits both COX-1 and COX-2 to differing degrees, as just one example, are well established for their most fundamental clinical application - reducing pain. However, much more specifically, these agents are also utilized for a range of applications including treating inflammation with/without the presence of joint damage, acute vs chronic pain afflicting patients with/as well as without chronic inflammation, as preventive approaches for both pain and inflammation following injury or surgery, and in conjunction with opioids when a simpler purely pain reducing approach is preferred. All of the aforementioned sub-indications, whether or not listed in official labeling, continue to be utilized in clinical practice and have continued to be so for a number of years now. Such examples are quite prevalent, and these "differing degrees" are perhaps just as common in other drugs preferred by clinicians.

In contradistinction to - and also in part because of - the growing awareness of the risks of systemic steroids, an array of other anti-inflammatory products have emerged to become part of the medical armamentarium that now threaten to replace systemic steroids for myriad clinical uses. While the current processes of replacing systemic steroids with these agents, and increasing the diversity and novelty of different applications for these agents, are currently highly fluid, in general these agents are all anti-inflammatory agents with relatively weak side effect profiles that, at their respective clinical points of contact and as a result of those side effect profiles as well as their safer-rather-than-sorry nature, are difficult from an efficacy standpoint to absolutely validate. However, in marked contrast to the historical 'mic drop,' wherein definitive local steroids redefined our use of systemic steroids, the possible emergent paradigm shift of these alternative agents used uniquely and/or at specific points of contact in place of systemic steroids, would argue better as the subject of consideration of the panel.

The Use of Steroids as a Treatment Option for Back Pain

1. Introduction to Back Pain and Steroids

Back pain is a common complaint among people of all ages, and many people generally chalk it up to stressful lifestyles or aging. What many people may not realize is that one of the most common treatments for back pain is a type of medication called steroids. Of course, steroids are found in therapeutic medication, not the performance-enhancing drugs that many athletes have been found to use in sporting events. While the use of any type of steroid may concern certain patients, it is quite safe. This paper will look at the use of steroids and their ability to treat pain – particularly the pain associated with a common medical condition and problem.

Steroids are a type of medication that is called a corticosteroid, which is different from the male hormone-related steroid compounds (they are indeed related, but they are completely different classes of compounds). These types of steroids are anti-inflammatory drugs, and they are delivered as medication to the body to help decrease the inflammation and handle the discomfort that happens once the body encounters various conditions. The painful symptoms come about thanks to the chemicals that are coursing through the body, just what is called prostaglandin. These chemicals are found in all of the organs of the body and also in the skin and any other structures that penetrate the body.

2. Types of Steroids Used for Back Pain

Back pain is an extreme discomfort that many individuals go through on a daily basis. It is known that almost up to 80 percent of Americans will experience some sort of back pain in their lives. The majority of all back pain cases are related to arthritis, muscle strains, and ligament "wearing." This pain almost always falls within the category of being acute pain. Acute pain can last anywhere from several days to weeks but generally goes away after a prescribed amount of time. Subacute pain is a kind of acute pain and might terminate on its own but may recur every now and then. Every now and then, back pain may turn chronic. This is when an individual's back pain does not go away and occurs on an everyday basis.

The use of steroids as a treatment option for back pain is that it is only for short-term use when acute pain does not go away. Other than back pain, other reasons for short-term use of oral steroids are joint pain, inflammation of the stomach and intestines, gout, acute osteoarthritis, and severe skin problems. Long-term use of oral steroids may be used for severe autoimmune diseases and should be in close relation with a doctor.

3. Mechanism of Action of Steroids in Back Pain Relief

The corticosteroids are chemically distinct from the anabolic steroids, which are used to enhance muscle mass and strength. Corticosteroids have diverse actions. They affect metabolism of glucose, reduce swelling, and stabilize the membranes of all body cells. Corticosteroids also reduce the production of inflammatory chemicals. As a treatment, these powerful drugs are used for a variety of conditions, including bone marrow transplantation, inflammation, anemia, and herpes. Corticosteroids have the medical benefit of relieving pain, itchiness, and redness. They may be used in oncology, ophthalmology, and many other fields of medicine.

The location of the final corticosteroid effect involves partition in the cell membrane, due to the low water solubility of corticosteroids, and then they diffuse into the cytoplasmic membrane of the cell. They then combine with corticosteroid receptors inside cells. As a result, various enzymes are synthesized, most notably lipocortin. Lipocortin inhibits phospholipase A2. It has been discovered that phospholipase A2 occupies all the known intracellular targets and initiates the cascade that leads to inflammation; phospholipase A2 is needed for all forms of inflammation in cells. Corticosteroids block the actions of phospholipase A2. Since inflammation was directly related to phospholipids, suppression of the phospholipase A2 pathway by corticosteroids shed light on its mechanism of action. This explains how corticosteroids reduce inflammation involved in allergy, arthritis, and various skin rashes.

4. Effectiveness of Steroids for Short-Term Back Pain Relief

Although steroids do show some effectiveness in treating pain and inflammation, there are only a few indications where the use of these corticosteroids is appropriate, and you should always consult your doctor prior to considering their use. Patients with a prior history of stroke, infection, or clotting of veins should avoid using steroids. The presence of various medical conditions such as high blood pressure, diabetes, infection, or ulcers may interfere with steroid usage and may influence the conditions upon which steroids can be used. Steroids for injection are quite common, and you may have used them for different types of pains.

Steroids are a group of medications that are often used to treat a variety of pain conditions. Corticosteroids are a form of steroid. performed an evidence-based review of the effectiveness of specific injection therapies for the lumbar spine in persons with chronic low back pain (LBP). A systematic review of the literature was performed to assess the use of injection therapies as compared to a control treatment for LBP, sciatica, and spinal stenosis. Only randomized controlled studies (RCTs) were used, and validated outcome measures of pain analysis were improvement in pain, decrease in pain, or decrease or discontinuation of medication, injection, or other medical services. The analysis of the published articles was limited to the lumbar region to evaluate the effectiveness of injection therapies.

5. Side Effects and Risks Associated with Steroid Use for Back Pain

No treatment is without potential risks, and the use of steroids to manage back pain is no different. While steroids can alleviate symptoms, they can also produce a wide range of potential side effects that diminish their value. For some, the trade-offs are favorable, but for others, their direct effects on health make them a less attractive alternative. Short-term side effects, including insomnia, irritation, nervousness, and even pain at the injection site, are common, though temporary.

The longer a patient uses the steroids, the more profound and permanent the effects might be. Patients who have been prescribed longer-term use of steroids might see unhealthy changes in their hands and fingers. Cranial swelling, known as cranial pressure, can increase uneasiness along the optic nerve, which could result in a reduction in the field of vision. Any symptoms of swelling in the optic nerve may be more evident in cases of pressure on the nerves or in the case of existing glaucoma. Patients should discuss the details of their prescribed treatments in order to make a decision that is most likely to meet their needs with their caregiver.

6. Comparison of Steroids with Other Treatment Options for Back Pain

Two complications can arise when the results of steroid therapy are compared with the results of other treatment methods. First, there may be differences in the initial severity of the disease, suggesting that the more severe diseases should have had the greatest benefit from the treatment, whereas it also may be the most difficult to help. Second, the chronic nature of the spine affects the number of times patients are needed to seek further surgery, so that conditions such as the use of steroid as pain relief can be blurred. For a valid comparison between steroid administration and bed rest with or without exercise treatment, two similar patient groups are treated without the administration of steroid. True comparison should also be randomized with a clinically similar group of patients in each treatment. At present, there is no final answer to these concerns, and the physician must guide the patient based on reasonable evidential matter.

7. Guidelines and Recommendations for the Use of Steroids in Back Pain Management

There are guidelines on the use of epidural steroid injections, particularly for radiculopathy. For other uses, there are only recommendations, such as for acute non-radicular back pain, where the North American Spine Society (NASS) advises not to use epidural injections, or the American Society of Regional Anesthesia and Pain Medicine for chronic non-radicular back pain, where they recommend against the use of epidural steroid injections. These guidelines/recommendations are often from pain societies and/or interventional pain physicians, which implies that their main argument is the healthcare costs.

For sciatic pain, European clinical guidelines are more permissive, enabling the family doctor to be less dependent on the interventional specialist. For peripheral facial palsy in children, the use of steroids does not come under scrutiny, especially in combination with antiviral agents. The effect of the use of steroids through oral intake or injection in any spinal region may lead to avascular necrosis, even the softest steroid, methylprednisolone. Since the use of steroids in the spine is off-label, family doctors as well as interventional specialists need to consider the unintended effects or complications more frequently.

8. Future Research Directions in Steroid Use for Back Pain

Identification of subgroups most likely to benefit from steroids is the ultimate goal. Currently, clinical trials do not account for this variability and so are not capable of answering these important questions. For individuals likely to respond, combination treatment strategies equating different etiologic diagnoses to potential suppressors of symptom generation and methods for removing temporally protective mechanisms may maximize the long-term benefits of a steroid. However, identifying responder subgroups should probably be the first step. Finally, of paramount importance is identifying subgroups for whom steroid injection is either of no utility or a net detriment. Stimulating research in these areas and in the refinement of new and existing depot forms will permit judicious use of corticosteroids in the ongoing management of low back pain.

In summary, when corticosteroids are well-centered within a treatment paradigm, they can add significant benefit to various dimensions of the symptomatic experience of low back pain. Importantly, benefits accrue to patients and healthcare providers alike. Such extra-time-related benefits are particularly well-suited to a modern healthcare system calling for cost-effective models of pain management. The more relevant question involving steroid injection for low back pain, then, is probably not if they work, but for whom, in both subacute and chronic stages of suffering.

www.ingramcontent.com/pod-product-compliance
Lightning Source LLC
Chambersburg PA
CBHW061936270726
48660CB00007BA/2932